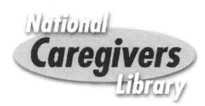

Caregiver's Workbook

Checklists and Worksheets for Family Caregivers

2nd Edition

by Ronald L. Moore

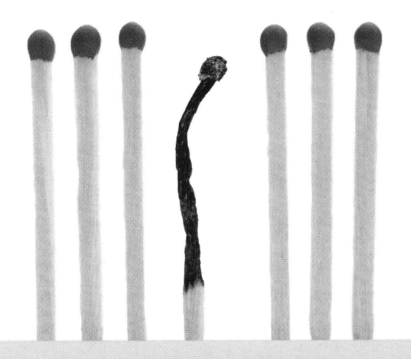

Caregiving can be one of the most emotionally traumatic, physically draining, mentally taxing and financially worrisome parts of an adult's life.

THIS WORKBOOK HELPS FAMILIES COPE

This workbook is a resource of:

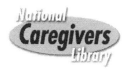

For free access to additional resources, please visit: **www.CaregiversLibrary.org**

Table of Contents

Introduction

Caregiving is never easy, but there are many things you can do to ease the burden.

Unfortunately, most caregivers simply aren't aware of the vast number of resources that are available to them – everything from government programs that can help pay for care to geriatric case managers who can perform assessments and arrange for necessary services. But accessing caregiving resources is only part of the problem. Many caregivers just don't know where to begin.

Caregiving is a process, not an event.

Throughout the process, caregivers take on a variety of roles. Some begin by performing everyday chores like cooking meals and driving a loved one to medical appointments and progress to assisting with personal activities like bathing, grooming, and dressing.

Along the way, caregivers may find themselves taking on responsibilities in many other areas, including arranging for medical treatment and managing medications; paying bills and managing financial affairs; and handling legal, housing, and insurance matters. The sheer number of tasks that caregivers perform can be overwhelming.

That's where this book comes in. The *Caregiver's Workbook* is filled with checklists, worksheets, and forms that can help make your caregiving responsibilities a little more manageable — a little easier. Inside, you'll find checklists to help you determine how much assistance your loved one needs; forms to help you evaluate nursing facilities, home health workers, and other services; and worksheets to help you organize and keep track of your loved one's important paperwork.

Use this book as a workbook. Write in it. Take notes in it. Use it to keep information and to refer to new chapters as you move through the caregiving process. And, while the book is copyrighted, there are several helpful forms within it that have been clearly marked as ones that you may make copies of so you can use them on an ongoing basis. We simply remind you to make copies only for your own, personal, non-commercial use.

The *Caregiver's Workbook*, however, is only one of many valuable resources from the National Caregivers Library. So while caregiving is never easy, we hope that tools like this *Caregivers Workbook* and the plethora of free resources available at **www.CaregiversLibrary.org** can simplify the process and help point you in the right direction; giving you information and support to help you provide your loved one with the best possible care.

NOTES

DATE OF ENTRY	A NOTE page will appear on every other page throughout this book. You may use this space to provide a written record of your on-going care for your loved one. Enter the date of each entry you make in the space provided on the left.

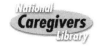

Who we are

The *Caregivers Workbook* is a resource of the National Caregivers Library and MetaMD, LLC.

Caregiving can be one of the most emotionally traumatic, physically draining, mentally taxing, and financially worrisome parts of an adult's life. **Our mission is to help caregivers**:

- Learn more about the process of caregiving.
- Get help managing their fears and concerns.
- Obtain information on, and access to, community resources, home health, caregiving-related products, health care, long-term care, housing, and financial and legal planning.

The National Caregivers Library is one of the largest sources of tools and information for caregivers and seniors in the country. Most of its resources are available to caregivers for free through alliances with professionals, businesses and other organizations who serve seniors and their caregivers with a variety of products and services.

Our web-based library, www.CaregiversLibrary.org consists of hundreds of useful articles, forms, checklists and links to external resources. It is organized into logical categories that address key needs of caregivers and their loved ones. Our website has been recognized by:

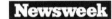

THE WALL STREET JOURNAL.   **Newsweek**   **Kiplinger**.com

Tools for employers. It provides tools to help employers understand the impact of caregiving on their people and on the organization itself. It provides tools to help identify the organizational costs of working caregivers and ways to analyze, justify, develop and implement Caregiving and Eldercare programs to help employees.

Caregiving Ministries™ provides resources for clergy, church leaders and their member caregivers including tools and support for starting care related ministry programs. We encourage the exchange of ideas and programs that minister to those in need. Our resources help faith organizations better understand the needs of their members and communities and help accelerate the creation and implementation of care ministries by shortening the "research and study" process.

Our Mission and Business. MetaMD's mission is to improve healthcare through education.

Recognizing the importance of family caregivers and the need to support them, MetaMD offers the resources of www.CaregiversLibrary.org for free for individual and family use.

In addition, we provide physician, clinician and patient education and training through preceptorships, seminars, one-to-one professional training and interactive patient education. MetaMD is nationally known for its interactive, educational programs for parents of newborns. These programs are used in Neonatal Intensive Care Units (NICU) and Labor & Delivery Departments in major hospitals across the country. For more information, visit www.NewParentEducation.com.

To learn how MetaMD can help your organization, call 804-327-1111.

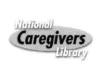

8

NOTES

DATE OF ENTRY	

Chapter 1: Taking Stock

Whether you have recently taken on the role of caregiver or you've been providing informal care for years, now is an excellent time to assess (or reassess) your caregiving situation. The questions in this section will help you (1) uncover the information you need to make wise decisions, (2) marshal the necessary resources and (3) create an Action Plan. This discovery process will help insure you are being both efficient and effective in providing the best possible care.

Maybe you weren't prepared to be a caregiver but an event or crisis placed you in the role. Or perhaps you assumed the responsibility incrementally, doing a little more of this or that over the years. Regardless of the situation, if you've provided care to a loved one for some time, you may feel as familiar with the ins and outs of his or her daily needs as your own.

Anticipate Future Needs

You may have grown so used to day-to-day requirements that you've been unable to give much thought to the future. What will your loved one's needs be in a few months? A year? How much additional assistance will be necessary? How will his or her condition change? What will change financially? Also consider what legal measures will need to be in place and what changes in living circumstances might prove necessary.

By systematically thinking through the situation, you might find new resources and opportunities to make caregiving a little easier, and be better able to anticipate new challenges. The forms and questions in this section can help you take a fresh look.

NOTES

DATE OF ENTRY	

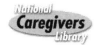

Caregiver's Assessment Worksheet

After completing both parts of this Worksheet, review your responses. Use the **Problem-Solving Worksheet** (later in this chapter) to write down the steps you want to take, based on your review.

Part I: About Your Care Recipient

Use this form to assess how much help your loved one needs, and in which areas. How has this changed during the past 3 to 6 months? **Use the following scale to classify the ability level.**

A = Accomplishes independently B = Needs some help C = Needs a great deal of help

Activity	Ability	What has changed recently?
1. Bathing		
2. Dressing		
3. Grooming		
4. Using the toilet		
5. Eating a nutritious diet		
6. Getting out of bed or chair		
7. Walking		
8. Taking medications and following medical instructions		
9. Using the telephone		
10. Shopping		
11. Preparing Meals		
12. Transportation (to doctor, etc.)		
13. Managing money		
14. Doing laundry		
15. Doing light housework		
16. Other:		
17. Other:		
18. Other:		
19. Other:		
20. Other:		

NOTES

DATE OF ENTRY	

Note: If your care recipient has any "C" ratings or even several "B's" in 1 through 8 above, review their support systems carefully. If this person is not currently living with someone, it may be time to reevaluate that decision. If driving is an issue, see **Driving Assessment**, in this Chapter.

Physical Challenges

How do the following affect the person's ability to function? Rate as follows:

"A" for no effect "B" for some effect "C" for major affect

Limitation	Ability	What has changed recently?
Hearing		
Vision		
Perception		
Orientation		
Cognition		
Memory		
Grasping		
Reaching out		
Balance		
Strength		
Energy		
Bladder or bowel control		
Arthritis		
Hypertension		
Heart disease		
Diabetes		
Physical deformity		
Chronic sinusitis		
Depression		

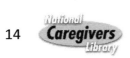

NOTES

DATE OF ENTRY	

Part II: About You, the Caregiver

1. How's your health? Good ❑   Fair ❑   Poor ❑

How is your role of caregiver affecting your health? Would you like to learn more about stress management techniques as a way of minimizing the effects of caregiving on your health?

2. Are you currently employed? Yes ❑ No ❑

If yes, have you talked with your company about policies and benefits available to working caregivers? (Note that many companies, particularly smaller ones, may not offer benefits.)

Do you understand your rights under the National Family and Medical Leave Act (FMLA)?

3. What types of services do you provide most often to your care receiver(s)?

   ❑ Physical—bathing, dressing, etc.

   ❑ Life management—paying bills, cooking, monitoring medications, shopping and errands, etc.

   ❑ Social—visits, telephone contact, transportation to social activities.

   ❑ Emotional support: (Describe) _____

   ❑ Financial: If so, have you budgeted for the expense as a part of your own financial plan? Would you like to know more about private insurance and government program coverage and reimbursements for your loved one? Would you like to learn more about long-term care insurance for yourself?

   ❑ Other: (Describe) _____

4. What is the average number of hours per week (or month) that you spend providing care? Where does this time come from? ❑ Work ❑ Family ❑ Friends & recreation ❑ All of these.

5. What kinds of changes in your home life have you and your family experienced as a result of you becoming a caregiver?

_____

_____

_____

16

NOTES

DATE OF ENTRY	

6. How have you and your family responded to these changes?

7. How do family members and friends support you in your caregiving activities? Are there additional ways in which you would like support from family members?

8. If you were no longer able to be the caregiver for the person you are caring for:

    A.   Who would be able to take over your responsibilities? _____

    B.   Have you spoken with this person about being a designated caregiver? Yes ❑ No ❑

    C.   Have you talked with the care recipient about what he or she would like to have happen in the event you can no longer carry on? Yes ❑ No ❑

    D.   Is everyone in the family aware of the care recipient's wishes and of the plan for what will happen if you are no longer able to be the caregiver? Yes ❑ No ❑

9. What community supports do you use? What barriers prevent you from using the supports NOT checked below? (Common barriers include lack of knowledge, time and organization.)

Support	Activity/Service Used	Barriers
❑ Friends		
❑ Neighbors		
❑ Clergy & church members		
❑ Social service agencies		
❑ Health care workers		
❑ Area Agency on Aging		
❑ Professional care managers		
❑ Caregiver or illness support group		

NOTES

DATE OF ENTRY	

10. To what extent do you experience the following feelings in your role as caregiver? Use the following scale to rank the frequency.

        A = Almost Never
        B = Sometimes
        C = = Frequently
        D = Almost Always

Feeling	Rank	Ways of Coping
Angry		
Anxious		
Appreciated		
Apprehensive		
Depressed		
Fearful		
Frustrated		
Fulfilled		
Guilty		
Lonely		
Overwhelmed		
Rewarded		
Tired		
Other feelings:		
Other feelings:		
Other feelings:		

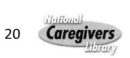

NOTES

DATE OF ENTRY	

Taking Care of Yourself

Caring for another person is the most difficult responsibility you will ever have. While many rewards come with caregiving, there are sacrifices, and demands may be high.

Because caregiving can be overwhelming, it's important to pace yourself. It's often difficult to know how long you'll need to provide care, or if your job will become more demanding over time. This job doesn't come with a job description!

Caring for your own needs is as important as taking care of the other person. If you are sick, or if you become physically or mentally exhausted, you can't care for someone else.

Common Feelings

It's normal for caregivers to feel sad or discouraged from time to time. Ignoring these feelings won't make them go away; it may even make them grow stronger.

- **If you feel sad:** Include some pleasant activities in your daily schedule. It can lift your spirits to listen to favorite music, spend a few moments enjoying the garden, or talk on the phone with a supportive friend.

- **If you feel discouraged:** Take one day at a time. Try to stay flexible and accept the things you can't change.

- **If you feel afraid:** Talk to someone about the worst thing that could happen and plan what you would do. Planning for the future will help reduce your fears about the "what ifs?"

- **If you feel angry:** Take a break and leave the situation if possible. A walk can help defuse your feelings. If you can't leave, stop and take a few deep deliberate breaths. It really does help. Focus your anger on the condition, not the person you care for.

- **If you feel guilty:** Give yourself credit for what you do well. Be realistic about what's possible and what isn't. Focus on one thing you want to do better and be specific. "If only I could make her eat" won't be as helpful as "I will slow down and make meal times more pleasant."

Talk to someone who can help you look at things more objectively, perhaps a friend, a fellow caregiver, or a professional counselor or your faith leader. Most communities have support groups you can join. These are usually organized around a particular disease or disability.

You might also call the Eldercare Locator at 1-800-677-1116 to find your local Area Agency on Aging that can provide information and referrals to local providers. Or, go online at http://www.eldercare.gov.

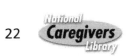

NOTES

DATE OF ENTRY	

Keep Yourself Physically and Mentally Healthy

Make sure you eat a healthy diet and get some form of exercise as often as possible. A brisk walk is a sure way to relieve stress.

- **Be honest with yourself**, friends and family about your needs.

- **Take a break.** Schedule time away on a regular basis. To maintain your own emotional and physical health it is absolutely necessary to get relief from your caregiving role.

- **Get enough rest.** If the person is awake at night and it's impossible for you to get a full night's sleep, you may need to consider in-home help during the night or an overnight respite stay. NOTE: Lack of sleep *for the caregiver* is a common reason that a loved one must enter a nursing home.

- **Eat properly.** A good diet will give you more energy. Even one diet improvement can make a big difference over a year's time.

- **Protect yourself against infection.** Wear disposable latex gloves if you will have contact with a body fluid.

- **Be kind to yourself.** Give yourself credit for the things you do well. Treat yourself to a small present when you're feeling low. Take time for a long, hot bath.

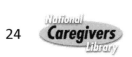

NOTES

DATE OF ENTRY	

Problem-Solving Worksheet

After reviewing the **Caregiver's Assessment** you performed in the first exercise, use this worksheet to help you attack any problems you identified.

Caregiving problems can be hard to solve. They are often complicated, involving many different, sometimes conflicting, factors. Consequences can affect other people's lives and health, usually people who are very important to you. They often involve unfamiliar, unexpected circumstances. And they almost always come with timetables, emotional baggage, and a load of stress.

Caregiving decisions are too important to make alone. Whenever possible, involve family members in the problem-solving process. Some family members may be able to see the situation more objectively than you, since you are likely to be stressed, harried and time-pressured. Other family members may be able to "protect" you by having that conversation about the trade-offs between independence and safety. Plus, multiple heads are better than one when brainstorming ideas and gathering information.

One essential person to include in the conversation, whenever possible, is the care receiver. His or her perspective on the problem may differ from everyone else's and must be given great weight out of love and respect. Involving the care recipient in decision-making, to the extent their capabilities permit, also will increase the likelihood of his or her agreeing to the decision itself.

Problem-Solving Is Easier When You Do It Step By Step

By breaking big decisions into these separate steps, you turn a potentially overwhelming problem into manageable pieces that can be accomplished one at a time. Indeed, the key to solving caregiving problems is dealing with them one at a time, starting with the most important one.

1. Identify the problem.
2. Get information.
3. Examine alternatives.
4. Make an action plan.
5. Give your decision time to work.
6. Evaluate how well it's working and adjust accordingly.

1. Identify the problem

Based on your review of the **Caregiver's Assessment**, what problems did you identify? Which one do you want to solve first? What makes it a problem? Who is affected (beyond the obvious folks)? What are the consequences if a solution cannot be found or put into effect?

NOTES

DATE OF ENTRY	

Write a description of the problem:

2. Get information

Your goal is to make a wise decision, based on as many facts as possible.

Four basic kinds of information about the care receiver are essential to consider: physical and functional information, psychological information, financial information, and social information.

Some key facts may come from outside sources, like your loved one's doctor, community agencies, or private professionals and services.

Other important factors include personal knowledge of the care recipient's beliefs and values. Checking with friends, neighbors and peripheral family members may uncover additional solutions or sources of help.

List key facts that relate to this problem and possible solutions.

3. Examine alternatives

Collect all the relevant ideas, information, and facts you can. Consider any and all of the ways you can to solve this problem. Encourage everyone to brainstorm ideas. At this stage, never prejudge the value or feasibility of an idea, regardless of its source.

Only after all the ideas are on the table should you weigh them against each other. What's the possible good from each one? The possible harm? How acceptable does it sound to the people it will most likely affect?

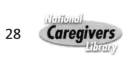

NOTES

DATE OF ENTRY	

Write the top three alternatives below:

	Alternative	Benefits	Challenges
1.			
2.			
3.			

The most successful alternative will probably be the one that:

- Has the fewest undesirable consequences.
- Appeals most strongly to the person most involved (usually the caregiver or receiver).
- Has the most support in the family.

The solution you arrive at may not be the perfect choice. But if it has risen to the top of the list, it is worth trying out and testing. Remember that a choice not to try anything different is a choice, too - and it could be a valid one.

4. Make an Action Plan

Make a list of which steps to take, in which order, and who should take them. Figure out which specific criteria will tell you whether or not the plan is working—and how much time you should allow to find out. Write down all these parts of your action plan, so you can measure its progress and effectiveness.

Goal:

_____

Action	Who	By When	Done
			❏
			❏
			❏
			❏
			❏

NOTES

DATE OF ENTRY	

5. Give Your Solutions Time to Work

No solution, even the best possible one, can change things overnight. So agree on a specific trial period after which you can evaluate how well your action plan works. How long should that trial period last? Long enough for the people involved in the new plan to start adjusting to it; long enough for potential or unexpected problems to surface, but short enough to correct mistakes early.

Make sure that everyone has a clear idea of what's expected of them throughout the trial period. Agree, too, that anyone who has doubts or conflicting ideas will put them aside throughout the trial period and devote their best efforts to making the plan succeed.

6. Evaluate Your Results and Adjust Accordingly

The family as a whole should define in advance what indicators will tell them that the plan is succeeding, failing, or falling somewhere in between.

As the trial period ends, evaluate the results against your criteria. The important thing here is not how the results compare to some abstract ideal, but whether the plan implemented makes things better than before.

- Has the plan actually changed things?

- Who's better off than before, and how?

- Who's worse off, and how?

- How much improvement has the plan brought about?

- Is there observable progress towards achieving the stated goals? Is there enough?

- Have unexpected obstacles arisen? Unexpected benefits?

- Should we give the plan more time? Or start working to change or replace it?

One of the biggest benefits of the trial and evaluation process is that it often redefines the problem—or, at least, gives you new information. With this new information at hand, the family can get together and go through the decision-making process again, setting new goals and testing different action plans on the basis of the added knowledge, information and experience this trial period has provided. As you do, you'll be moving closer and closer to better and more workable solutions.

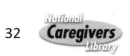

NOTES

DATE OF ENTRY	

Driving Assessment

As the population of individuals 65 years and older continues to increase in the United States— and because the physical changes that come with aging make driving more dangerous for the elderly—the issue of confronting elderly parents, relatives, and friends who are no longer safe drivers is a problem that will continue to grow.

It can be difficult to tell if your loved one has driving difficulties, but one of the most obvious signs includes excessive dents in his or her car. Don't depend solely on your loved one or his or her doctor to tell you about possible problems. Additionally, it doesn't make sense to rely solely on a state driving agency, as individuals with certain types of problems (e.g., slow reflexes) can still pass a driving test. Yet, if you are concerned about your loved one's driving, his or her doctor and the state agency are good places to gain useful information.

Unfortunately, but not surprisingly, it is very difficult to talk with a loved one about his or her driving; and it's even harder to ask that he or she no longer drive. Therefore, it is often easier to start by discussing the topic with a doctor who can assess your loved one's muscle strength, eyesight, reflexes, and general overall health. Additionally, you might want to find out about state-specific driving regulations and recommendations for impaired or elderly drivers.

If you decide that your loved one's driving is dangerous, approach the topic carefully. Remember that driving is linked to independence, so if you decide to approach your loved one, try to make a caring request (e.g., Dad, I've been a little concerned about your car because it has many dents and scratches on it) rather than a command (e.g., Dad, I think that you are too old to drive because you keep hurting the car). If you anticipate that your loved one will disagree with you in an extreme fashion, you might want to try video-taping him or her driving and showing the tape to your loved one. It may also help to have his or her doctor talk directly with your loved one about driving.

Regardless of who broaches the subject, it should be a person that your loved one is comfortable with, and it should be done in a respectful way. In many cases the discussion of your loved one's driving and possible alternative transportation options will be an ongoing conversation. During each conversation, be patient and firm. After all, your loved one may be coping with what he or she perceives as a loss of independence, but his or her safety and that of others is ultimately the most important issue.

If you are unsure about your loved one's driving, use the **Driving Assessment Checklist** on the next page to determine whether or not you may need to make alternative transportation arrangements.

NOTES

DATE OF ENTRY	

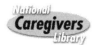

Driver Assessment Checklist

The following list can help you evaluate your loved one's ability to drive. Checking "yes" for multiple items suggests that you should talk with your loved one about his or her driving and look into alternative transportation options.

	YES	NO
1) A police officer has given your loved one a warning because of poor driving behavior.	❏	❏
2) Your loved one's record has accidents, close calls, violations, and/or minor collisions.	❏	❏
3) Driving makes your loved one nervous and anxious.	❏	❏
4) It is difficult for your loved one to look over his or her shoulder or to turn his or her head to the side to look before changing lanes.	❏	❏
5) Driving makes your loved one tired.	❏	❏
6) Your loved one has trouble climbing stairs or walking more than one block in a day.	❏	❏
7) Your loved one often becomes disoriented about where he or she is in relation to home.	❏	❏
8) Your loved one backs up after missing an exit.	❏	❏
9) Your loved one recovers slowly from the glare of oncoming headlights, streetlights, or other shiny objects while driving during the day or at night.	❏	❏
10) Your loved one has a difficult time seeing people, traffic signs, lane lines, or other objects around or on the road.	❏	❏
11) Your loved one often "misses" red lights or stop signs and as a consequence goes through them.	❏	❏
12) Your loved one backs into and over things such as curbs.	❏	❏
13) Passing cars frighten your loved one due to their noise or speed.	❏	❏
14) Other drivers tailgate or pass your loved one most of the time.	❏	❏
15) Your loved one has a difficult time with hand/foot coordination.	❏	❏

NOTES

DATE OF ENTRY	

16) Your loved one has mistaken the gas pedal for the brake.	❏	❏
17) Your loved one had a stroke, or has amyotrophic lateral sclerosis (ALS), dementia, epilepsy, multiple sclerosis, Parkinson's disease, seizure or sleep disorders, or uncontrolled diabetes that could affect his or her driving ability.	❏	❏
18) Your loved one takes medication for a prior stroke, or for amyotrophic lateral sclerosis (ALS), dementia, epilepsy, multiple sclerosis, Parkinson's disease, seizure or sleep disorders, or uncontrolled diabetes that could affect his or her driving ability.	❏	❏
19) Your loved one's driver's license was not checked when he or she turned age 70.	❏	❏
20) Your loved one's driver's license has not been checked every three years since he or she turned 70 (e.g., 73, 76, 79) or annually since he or she turned 80.	❏	❏
21) Your loved one fails to appreciate the frustration or irritation of other drivers in response to his / her own driving.	❏	❏

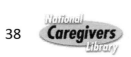

NOTES

DATE OF ENTRY	

Caregiver's Organizing System

Caregiving is hard enough without allowing yourself to be overwhelmed with papers, papers and more papers. Getting organized is a major time-saver. The process is simple: eliminate what you don't need, organize the things that you must keep, and put simple systems into place to keep things from getting out of control. Here are some suggestions for setting up "Command Central," a place to organize and keep track of the details of your caregiving situation.

Command Central can be as simple as a three-ring binder where you record information, monitor changes, and keep track of important contacts. Or it can be physical place: a table, a filing cabinet, or a desk in a quiet corner. Once you establish your spot, follow this tried and true procedure.

1. Know what to hold, and what to toss

Gather all related papers, prescriptions, plans, notes to yourself, forms, etc., at Command Central and weed through them. Ask yourself, "Do I really need this?" Get rid of it if the answer is "No." If the answer is "Maybe," put it in a holding bin or box to sort through later. Reasons to *eliminate* papers are:

- It's old or out of date.
- If you ever do need it, you can find it elsewhere.
- You can delegate or pass on the information.

2. Organize the remaining papers

Begin to categorize and prioritize what is left. Ask yourself, "What do I do with it? What categories and systems do I need in place?" Active documents are papers you might refer to in the next several weeks, and which need to be readily accessible. Set up folders and files for these "Actives." Make the labels match your "what-do-I-do-with-it" categories, e.g., Health Records, Insurance Reimbursement, Important Contacts, Action Plans, Community Services, etc. Items you may want to have handy include:

- A list of informal support networks, such as a neighbor who runs errands or a youth who shovels snow, chops wood or cuts the grass.

- Copies of your action plan(s) and records of family discussions.

- Services or support your loved one needs or wants.

- A list of your needs as a caregiver. This will give you something easy and specific to refer to when someone asks, "What can I do to help?"

- A running list of situations that need attention or changing.

- A plan for maintaining your own physical, mental, and financial well-being.

Inactive papers are those used infrequently. If at all possible, keep them away from Command Central in a spot where they are safe and accessible, but won't clutter your new system.

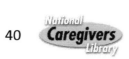

NOTES

DATE OF ENTRY	

3. Create an "in-box" procedure

Design a place for incoming information and mark it clearly. Everything goes into the box, no exceptions. Then schedule a routine time to process box contents. Decide whether to do it, file it, delegate it, delay it, or read it. This is the real secret of staying organized; don't let the piles pile up in the first place; deal with them regularly instead.

4. Create and distribute copies of critical documents and procedures to family members

Engineers know the importance of redundant systems, a second computer that kicks in if the first one fails, for example. Your caregiving systems are no less important. Who will step in if you get sick and can't perform? Will someone else know who to call and what to do? Capture and photocopy this information and distribute it to other key family members. This will save time and reduce risks in the event of an emergency. It will also provide someone else with a caregiving "blueprint" to follow if they fill in for you

(If this procedure is helpful, also see the **Document Organizer** in the chapter on *Legal Matters*).

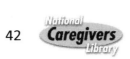

42

NOTES

DATE OF ENTRY	

Chapter 2: Home Care

If your loved one lives at home—or with you or another family member—the tools in this section can help you maintain a safe and comfortable environment while ensuring that he or she gets the best possible care.

To begin, here's a list of basic ideas for making the daily caregiving experience easier for you and your loved one.

- **Encourage independence.** Be a helper instead of a doer. Even if you can do things faster or better, encourage her to use the skills she still has. Skills that aren't used will be lost.

- **Personal care** (dressing, bathing, eating, using the toilet) is personal. Everybody does these activities differently. Try to use the same routines the person is used to.

- **Be flexible.** The person may not need a daily bath. They might prefer several small snacks rather than three larger meals every day.

- **Divide tasks into smaller steps.** If he can't shave on his own because his hand is unsteady, let him apply the lather and wash off with a cloth after he's been shaved.

- **Look for gadgets that increase independence.** For an unsteady person, long tongs or "reachers" make it easier to pick things up from the floor. It's possible to peel potatoes with one hand by using a special board with a nail sticking up to anchor the potato. Several good catalogs will give you many ideas. Search online or call your local Sears or J.C. Penney's and ask for a home health catalog.

- **Give praise for trying.** Especially when a person's abilities are limited, a sincere "well- done" is often appreciated.

- **Consider getting professional advice** to learn easier ways to help the other person. Nurses, home health aides, physical, occupational and speech therapists are trained to teach family members how to provide care in the home. Ask your doctor for a referral.

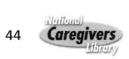

NOTES

DATE OF ENTRY	

Community Resources

While every community is different, most offer a variety of services that can lighten your caregiving load. Ask your faith leader or call 1-800-677-1116 to find your local Area Agency on Aging, which can provide referrals. Here is a list of the types of services that might be available in your area.

- **Adult Day Care/Adult Day.** Health and Social activities, therapies, health education and supervision are often provided in a group setting during the day in facilities such as churches, nursing homes, and community centers. Some centers provide transportation.

- **Adult Protective Services** will investigate possible abuse, neglect, exploitation, or abandonment and provide short-term emergency support services to adults in need of protection.

- **Case Managers or Geriatric Care Managers** can help develop a complete plan of services based on the individual's needs and provide follow-up to make sure that needed services are provided.

- **Environmental Modifications.** A person may be eligible for free modifications to the home that will increase independence and allow the person to stay in the home.

- **Health Screening** (typically for persons 60 and older) is available in some communities for general health assessment, limited physical examinations and some laboratory tests.

- **Mental Health Services** include evaluation, emergency, and outpatient treatment.

- **Minor Household Repairs** may be available if necessary for health and safety.

- **Respite Care** provides relief for caregivers of adults with disabilities, and can be arranged through home health agencies, Adult Family Homes, Adult Residential Care, social day care, nursing homes, family, friends, or volunteers.

- **Senior Meals** (if person or spouse is 60 or older) provides nutritious meals in a group setting or delivered to home-bound persons.

- **Transportation** may be available for medical and social services, meal programs, shopping and recreational activities.

Your community may have other services that aren't listed here. It may take some time to find out about all that is available, and what will be most helpful. The following worksheet can help you keep track of your conversations with these services.

(NOTE: You may want to make multiple copies of this form—one for each agency that you interview.)

NOTES

DATE OF ENTRY	

Community Services Interview Record

Feel free to make multiple copies of this form so you can keep a record of in-person and phone interviews with different service agencies.

(You are hereby granted permission to make multiple copies of this form for personal, non-commercial use only.)

Date: _____

Agency:_____

Address: _____

Phone:_____

Name/Title of Person Interviewed:

Are there eligibility requirements? What are they?

_____

_____

_____

_____

Is there an application process? What is required?

_____

_____

_____

_____

_____

_____

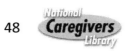

NOTES

DATE OF ENTRY	

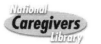

List services provided and any fees associated with those services.

_____

_____

_____

_____

_____

List payment acceptable methods. (Medicare, Medicaid, Medical Assistance, private insurance, other.)

_____

_____

_____

_____

Is there a sliding fee scale? What are the qualifications for a reduced rate?

_____

_____

_____

Is written information available? Is it being sent?

_____

_____

NOTES

DATE OF ENTRY	

Home Care Workers

If your loved one lives at home and you cannot be there to provide daily care a skilled or semi-skilled home care worker may provide a solution.

First, decide how much assistance your loved one needs with medication, bathing, dressing, cooking, housekeeping, transportation, or other daily activities. **The Caregivers Assessment Worksheet in Chapter 1** can help you make this determination.

- Hold a family meeting and consider the observations of other family members.

- Discuss these topics with your loved one. Ask what kind of assistance he or she thinks would be most helpful, emphasizing the shared goal of maximized independence.

- Ask your loved one's doctor to offer advice or make a recommendation.

Compare your loved one's requirements to the kind of care provided by the four categories of home care workers below:

1. **A housekeeper or chore worker** performs basic household tasks and light cleaning.

2. **A homemaker or personal care worker** provides personal care, meal planning, household management, and medication reminders.

3. **A companion or live-in** provides personal care, light housework, exercise, companionship, and medication reminders.

4. **A home health aide, certified nurse's assistant, or nurses' aide** provides personal care and helps with transfers, exercise, household services essential to health care, and medication assistance. Additional duties include reporting changes in your loved one's condition to an RN or therapist, and keeping medical records.

Once you've determined what kind of worker is best, use the following **Home Care Workers Questions** worksheet to help you evaluate different home care agencies, compare services, and hire the best help available.

NOTES

DATE OF ENTRY	

Home Care Workers Questions

When Hiring Help Through An Agency, Find Out:

- How long the agency has been in business.

- Is the agency JCAHO (Joint Commission on Accreditation of Healthcare Organizations) accredited and Medicare certified?

- Which services are covered by Medicare?

- What type of employee screening does the agency perform?

- Whether you or the agency will be responsible for paying the worker.

- Whether you or the agency is responsible for supervising the worker.

- What types of general and specialized training do the workers have?

- Whether the same person will care for your loved one each day.

- Who to call if the worker fails to show up.

- How the agency responds to emergency needs.

- How the agency handles complaints.

- What fees the agency charges and what types of care each fee covers.

- Whether the agency offers a sliding fee scale.

- How do the fees vary for care provided during nights, weekends, or holidays?

- The minimum and maximum hours of service per worker provided.

- Any limitations on tasks performed or times of day when services are furnished.

- Whether the workers are agency employees or independent contractors.

- What insurance coverage does the agency AND its workers have? (worker's comp, general liability, malpractice, etc.)

- Are all taxes covered by the fees paid?

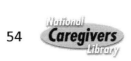

NOTES

DATE OF ENTRY	

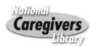

Certain information and guidelines should always be established up front. This can occur through face-to-face interviews with individual workers or when conferencing with the agency.

- Have a full and complete discussion of your loved one's needs.

- Get a full account of the applicant's experience and his or her expectations, or a comprehensive review of the agency's training requirements and certification standards.

- Explain what you want done and how you would like it done, keeping in mind that the worker is there to care for your loved one and not the rest of the family.

- Be clear about the worker's salary, the pay period, and reimbursement for gas, groceries, and other expenses.

- Discuss policies for vacations, holidays, absences, lateness, and termination.

- Talk about your loved one's dietary restrictions. Provide a list of contacts in case of an emergency, review security precautions and keys, and discuss your loved one's medication requirements.

- If the worker lives in the home, make sure that he or she has living quarters that give everyone the maximum amount of privacy possible.

- If public transportation isn't available and your loved one isn't eligible for free or low- cost transportation, try to hire someone who drives, since this can save you substantial amounts of money in taxi or commercial van ride fares. If the home care worker is going to drive your car, be sure to check with your insurance company concerning any limitations on your policy.

NOTES

DATE OF ENTRY	

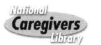

Caregiver's Log

NOTE: Make multiple copies of this 2-page log before writing. Save this original as a blank.
(You are hereby granted permission to make multiple copies of this form for personal, non-commercial use only.)

Once you've hired in-home help, you'll need a way to coordinate the care your loved one receives. This is especially important if different workers will be providing care during different times of the day or week. This **Caregiver's Log** is a simple form for each caregiver to record activities, changes in your loved one's daily condition or any RED FLAGS that need immediate attention.

These forms should be reviewed daily and shared with appropriate parties. Keep these logs in a central folder or 3-ring binder.

Use copies of this form to monitor daily changes and help with communication among care providers working in shifts.

Caregiver Name:_____

Organization (if any): _____

Phone: _____

Day and Date: _____

Hours : _____

Special activates or changes Noted:

RED FLAGS:

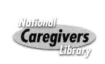

NOTES

DATE OF ENTRY	

Food:	Amount	Time	Comment
Activities:	Duration	Time	Comment
Medication: (see note***)	Dose	Time	Comment

(*You may want to use the Weekly Medicine Record in Chapter 4)**

Based on your observations of the care recipient, rate the following from 1–10, with 1 being the lowest and 10 the highest.

Pain & Discomfort:	1	2	3	4	5	6	7	8	9	10
Energy Level:	1	2	3	4	5	6	7	8	9	10
Sleep Pattern:	1	2	3	4	5	6	7	8	9	10
Nausea/Constipation:	1	2	3	4	5	6	7	8	9	10

Other Observations:

_____

_____

_____

_____

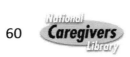

NOTES

DATE OF ENTRY	

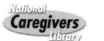

Home Safety Checklist

You might not have to make extensive modifications to the home to ensure your loved one's safety. There are some simple steps you can follow to create a safer caregiving environment.

Unfortunately, we often wait until an accident happens before we make changes. Act now to provide a safer home. The steps you take to improve safety at home will reduce the chance of serious injury and give you greater peace of mind.

Use this checklist as a starting point for conducting your own safety "walk-through." The questions are designed to help you isolate current problems and recognize potential hazards.

	YES	NO
Throughout the home:		
Is the lighting sufficient?	❏	❏
Are lamp, extension, and telephone cords placed out of flow of traffic?	❏	❏
Are light switches located near the entrance of each room?	❏	❏
Are cords out from beneath furniture and rugs and carpeting?	❏	❏
Are there enough outlets to handle all cords without overloading?	❏	❏
Are all small rugs and runners slip resistant?	❏	❏
Are there smoke detectors on every floor?	❏	❏
Is there an emergency plan?	❏	❏
Does your loved one have a personal alert system?	❏	❏
In the Kitchen:		
Are towels, curtains, and other flammables kept away from the range?	❏	❏
Are appliance cords located away from the sink or range?	❏	❏
Is there good, even lighting over the stove, sink, and countertop areas, especially where food is sliced and cut?	❏	❏

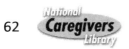

NOTES

DATE OF ENTRY	

In the bedroom:

Are lamps or light switches within reach of the bed? ❏ ❏

Is there a phone within reach of the bed? ❏ ❏

Are there loose rugs or runners in the areas around the bed? ❏ ❏

Are phone and lamp cords tucked in a safe place? ❏ ❏

Are there enough "night lights" to enable your loved one to see without overheads? ❏ ❏

In the bathroom:

Are bathtubs and showers equipped with non-skid mats, abrasive strips, or non-slick surfaces? ❏ ❏

Do bathtubs and showers have grab bars and/or benches as needed? ❏ ❏

Is the water temperature 120 degrees or lower? ❏ ❏

In stairways and hallways:

Are light switches located at the top and bottom of stairs? ❏ ❏

Are exits and passageways kept clear? ❏ ❏

Is carpeting fixed? ❏ ❏

Are steps even and of equal height? ❏ ❏

Do steps allow secure footing? ❏ ❏

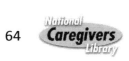

NOTES

DATE OF ENTRY	

Help with Home Modification

Once you've evaluated the home, you may find you need to make some modifications to increase safety. If you, your friends, or relatives are unable to do the project yourselves, it's worth it to look into local home modification and repair programs. Consider contacting a **Certified Aging-in-Place Specialist** about the best ways to help your loved one remain in his/her home.

Where to find help. Often, such programs can be located through your local Area Agency On Aging, State Agency On Aging, State Housing Finance Agency, Department of Public Welfare, Department Of Community Development, Senior Centers, or Independent Living Centers.

If you decide to hire a private contractor, make certain that he or she is reliable. Older people are prime targets for con artists and fraud. Be especially wary of door-to-door repair salespeople. Consider taking these steps:

- Get recommendations from friends who have had similar projects completed.

- Make sure that the contractor is licensed and bonded.

- Try to get bids from several contractors.

- Ask for references from previous customers—*and check them out*. Ask to see some of the contractor's completed projects.

- Check with your local Better Business Bureau or your city/county Consumer Affairs Office

- **Insist on a written agreement that thoroughly describes the work to be done, the materials to be used, the schedule of payments to be made, and a timeframe for completing the work – including penalties for the contractor not completing the work as promised. Also have the contractor agree in writing that he/she is responsible for:**

    o Cleaning the worksite daily; doing a final cleanup and removal of debris; providing proof of insurance (worker's compensation, liability, performance bonds, etc.) before _any_ money is paid; paying all taxes, including payroll taxes, and; making timely payments to sub-contractors and those working as independent contractors.

- Pay only a small down payment, followed by specific progress payments. Typically, progress payments are made once the materials are brought to your home, at one or more logical stages of the project (depends on the size, nature and duration of the project), and a final payment is made *after* the job is completed and inspected to your satisfaction.

- Have the agreement reviewed by a lawyer if it is very complicated.

- Make the final payment only after the project is completed. **DO NOT MAKE A FINAL PAYMENT IF THERE ARE ANY ISSUES TO BE CLEARED UP OR WORK REMAINING TO BE DONE.**

NOTES

DATE OF ENTRY	

Chapter 3: Choosing a Care Facility

While most people prefer to live at home as long as possible, age, infirmity, or illness often make home living impractical or unsafe. Generally, facilities at the beginning of the following list offer only basic residential services, such as housekeeping. In contrast, facilities at the end offer round-the-clock medical services and other specialized types of care.

Independent Living Facilities or Retirement Communities allow individuals to live in their own house, apartment, or condominium. They often offer smaller services such as social activities, meals, or housekeeping for an additional fee.

Group Homes provide an independent living environment with only minimal services. Group Homes differ from Independent Living Facilities in that the individual usually co-owns or rents the home with a group of individuals who share the common areas of the living environment.

Congregate Care Facilities offer private living quarters with additional services, including transportation, housekeeping, or religious services. Like retirement communities, these residential communities offer the individual a chance to live around other seniors.

Assisted Living Facilities provide care for individuals who require help with personal needs (e.g., bathing and grooming). They also offer meals, housekeeping, and administration of medications.

Nursing Homes offer 24-hour medical care under a doctor's supervision. They also provide room, meals, assistance with daily living, and recreational activities for residents. Most residents in these homes have physical or mental impairments that prevent independent living.

Continuing Care Retirement Communities accept seniors while they are still independent, and then provide an expanding range of services—including professional nursing care—as needed.

In addition to the above facilities, there are some residential care settings that are not easily categorized. Be sure to look into the specific types of facilities available in your loved one's area for more information.

Regardless of the level of care that your loved one needs or the types of facilities visited, **Questions for Assisted Living** and the **Nursing Home Checklist** can help you record information and compare impressions of different facilities. You may want to make copies for each facility you visit and evaluate several different facilities before making a final decision.

NOTES

DATE OF ENTRY	

Questions For Assisted Living

Refer to these questions for each assisted living facility you and your loved one visit. This will help you select the best possible place.

Keep in mind that the term "assisted living" encompasses a wide range of care and services, and that each state applies the term differently. Remember, too, that every community is unique. Some of the items below may not apply to the facility you are considering, and your loved one may not even require such services.

General Impressions

How often are activities in the community scheduled? What staff members are included?

Who develops and supervises recreational activities? What is this person's background? Do residents have input into activities offered?

Can residents walk on the grounds? Are there protected/enclosed walking areas for residents with dementia?

How are religious/spiritual needs met? Is there transportation to church or synagogue? Are there rooms and arrangements for worship programs in the facility?

Are there excessive or very unpleasant odors? (Note: Expect some unpleasant odors. What is important is whether they are excessive or caused by lack of cleaning, or neglect of residents.)

Evaluate the general level of cleanliness – in public areas, residents' rooms, bathrooms, dining rooms, kitchen, parking lot, etc.

NOTES

DATE OF ENTRY	

Meals

Sample a few meals. How does the food taste? If your loved one has special dietary needs, describe them and ask how those needs can be met. Ask to see a printed menu for the month.

What times are meals served?

What happens if a resident is late, misses a meal, or refuses a meal? Is the answer different if a resident is confused?

What if a resident wants to skip a meal? Is the answer different if a resident is confused?

Can residents request to have trays delivered to their rooms? Is there any additional charge?

If a resident doesn't like a meal, what are the alternatives?

Are snacks available at any time? What kinds of snacks are available?

Does a nutritionist or dietitian review meals and special diets? If yes, how often?

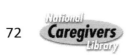

NOTES

DATE OF ENTRY	

Safety/Choice

Facilities vary with regard to the extent of protection they offer residents and may use negotiated risk agreements or contracts when issues of safety and choice arise. Ask the facility whether it uses any form of negotiated risk agreements. If they do, they should explain what they mean by the terms they use and how they use such agreements.

What safety measures protect residents from wandering?

What is the policy concerning personal property being stolen?

What if residents want an exception to a policy, e.g. signing in and out, smoking, or eating foods that are not on a prescribed diet? Is the answer different if a resident is confused?

Are background checks performed on all staff? What kind?

Which doors of the facility are locked and when? Are exit doors alarmed?

Are there safety locks on the windows?

Are there call bells in each room and bathroom? How often are they checked to be sure they are working?

Is there a fire emergency plan? Are there emergency sprinklers? When were they last checked? Are fire drills held? Are emergency plans publicly displayed?

Is the floor covering of the facility made of a nonskid material?

NOTES

DATE OF ENTRY	

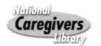

Facility Initiated Discharge

Answers to these questions will help you clarify a facility's ability to care for people with health and behavior conditions that are more difficult to manage.

What are reasons for discharge?

Is there an internal appeal process? What is it?

How many days notice is given and to whom?

How does the facility assist you if they proceed with discharge?

NOTES

DATE OF ENTRY	

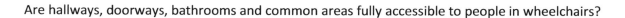

Accessibility

Are hallways, doorways, bathrooms and common areas fully accessible to people in wheelchairs?

If it is a multi-floor facility, what are the safety arrangements for escape in case of fire for people in wheelchairs?

Special Care Units

This section is directed to family members or other interested persons, because it would be unusual for the person who needs a special care unit to be asking these questions. These questions should be asked in addition to previous questions.

Is there a separate area specifically for people with dementia?

How do services in the special care unit differ from services in the rest of the facility?

What is the difference in staff training? What is the staff-to-resident ratio?

Do residents go out-of-doors regularly? How often? Where do they go? Does anyone go with them?

How do they ensure that residents are getting proper nutrition? Are finger foods available? Do they offer decaffeinated drinks throughout the day?

NOTES

DATE OF ENTRY	

Look at a calendar of activities. Do they appear appropriate for the resident?

Do the residents on the unit seem as disabled as the prospective resident?

What is the facility's policy on restraints, both chemical and physical?

Is there space to walk around on the unit?

What are the room arrangements?

If there will be a roommate, does he/she have any habits or mannerisms that would be difficult for the prospective resident to handle, e.g. staying up late at night, yelling, going through personal possessions of others?

When rooms are shared, what does the facility do if problems such as those in the previous question arise?

What is the cost difference between special care and regular units?

NOTES

DATE OF ENTRY	

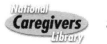

Nursing Home Checklist

Facility Name: Contact Person and Phone:

Address: Date Visited:

Basic Information	YES	NO
Accepting new patients	❏	❏
Medicare certified	❏	❏
Medicaid certified	❏	❏
Waiting period for admission	❏	❏
The home and the current administrator are licensed	❏	❏
The home conducts background checks on all staff	❏	❏
The home has Special Services Units	❏	❏
The home has Abuse Prevention Training	❏	❏
Number of beds in each category available to you:		

For parts two through five, give the nursing home a grade from one to five. One is poor, five is best.
The nursing home with the highest score is likely the best choice.

Quality of Care

1) Residents can make choices about their daily routine.	1	2	3	4	5
2) The interaction between staff and patient is warm and respectful.	1	2	3	4	5
3) The home is easy for friends and family to visit.	1	2	3	4	5
4) The nursing home meets your cultural, religious, or language needs.	1	2	3	4	5
5) The nursing home smells and looks clean and is well lighted.	1	2	3	4	5
6) The home maintains comfortable temperatures.	1	2	3	4	5
7) The resident rooms have personal articles and furniture.	1	2	3	4	5
8) The public and resident rooms have comfortable furniture.	1	2	3	4	5
9) The nursing home and its dining room are generally quiet.	1	2	3	4	5
10) Residents may choose from a variety of activities that they enjoy.	1	2	3	4	5
11) The nursing home welcomes outside volunteer groups.	1	2	3	4	5
12) The nursing home has outdoor areas for residents' use.	1	2	3	4	5
OTHER:	1	2	3	4	5

Quality of Care Score = _____

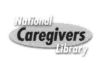

82

NOTES

DATE OF ENTRY	

Quality of Life

1) The facility corrected any Quality of Care deficiencies that were in the State Inspection Report.   1 2 3 4 5

2) Residents may continue to see their personal physician.   1 2 3 4 5

3) Residents are clean, appropriately dressed, and well groomed.   1 2 3 4 5

4) The staff responds quickly to calls for help.   1 2 3 4 5

5) The administrator and staff seem comfortable with each other and with the residents.   1 2 3 4 5

6) Residents have the same caregivers on a daily basis.   1 2 3 4 5

7) There are enough staff at night and on weekends or holidays to care for each resident.   1 2 3 4 5

8) The home has an arrangement for emergency situations with a nearby hospital.   1 2 3 4 5

9) The Family and Residents' Councils are independent from the nursing home's management.   1 2 3 4 5

10) Meetings to develop the Care Plan are held at times that are easy for residents and their family members to attend.   1 2 3 4 5

OTHER: 1 2 3 4 5

Quality of Life Score = _____

Nutrition Information

1) The home corrected any deficiencies in these areas that were on the recent survey.   1 2 3 4 5

2) There are enough staff to assist each resident who requires help with eating.   1 2 3 4 5

3) The food smells and looks good and is served at proper temperatures   1 2 3 4 5

4) Residents are offered choices of food at mealtimes.   1 2 3 4 5

5) Resident weight is routinely monitored.   1 2 3 4 5

6) There are water pitchers and glasses on tables in the rooms.   1 2 3 4 5

7) Staff helps residents to drink if they are not able to do so on their own.   1 2 3 4 5

8) Nutritious snacks are available during the day and evening.   1 2 3 4 5

9) The dining room environment encourages residents to relax, socialize, and enjoy their food.   1 2 3 4 5

OTHER: 1 2 3 4 5

Nutrition Score = _____

NOTES

DATE OF ENTRY	

Safety

1) There are handrails in hallways and grab bars in bathrooms.	1	2	3	4	5
2) Exits are clearly marked.	1	2	3	4	5
3) Spills and other accidents are cleaned up quickly.	1	2	3	4	5
4) Hallways are free of clutter and are well-lighted.	1	2	3	4	5
5) There are enough staff to help move residents quickly in an emergency.	1	2	3	4	5
6) The nursing home has smoke detectors and sprinklers.	1	2	3	4	5
OTHER:	1	2	3	4	5

Safety Score = _____

TOTAL SCORE for this facility - _____

NOTES FROM VISIT:

NOTES

DATE OF ENTRY	

Adjusting to Long-Term Care

Once you've found the right care facility, you'll probably have to help your loved one through an adjustment period. Adjusting emotionally to a long-term care facility can be difficult. After all, living in your own home is always easier than learning the rules and norms of another place. Additionally, it is often harder to maintain important possessions due to facility regulations. For instance, moving into a long-term care facility often means giving up a beloved pet.

For these reasons, you loved one may feel a range of emotions about the move, including anger, confusion, depression, disorientation, and grief.

These emotions are all normal. Help your loved one to understand this and encourage him or her to work through the negative emotions, to "keep" a piece of his or her past living environment, and to adjust to the new location.

You can help your loved one to do these things by being involved in the moving process. Remind your loved one that the new rules are for his or her safety, but that these rules still allow him or her to have a "home," whether it is an apartment or a bed in a shared room.

Find out what is important to your loved one and help him or her find a way to remember or keep these memories, possessions, or people in his or her life. In doing so you may need to be inventive by doing things like:

- Creating a special place, whether it be a bench outside or a decorated wall in your loved one's room

- Finding a home for his / her pet with a neighbor / friend who will allow the pet to visit your loved one

- Helping your loved one to write and/or read letters from family, friends, and neighbors

- Learning about the new residence with your loved one

- Taking pictures of important possessions and hanging these in prominent places in the new residence

Most importantly, help your loved one to understand and remember that moving was necessary for his or her safety and health, and that although the new surroundings are different; there are many positive aspects of each living environment.

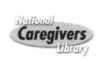

NOTES

DATE OF ENTRY	

Chapter 4: Medical Caregiving

While caregiving can involve many different jobs and roles, almost all caregivers find themselves dealing with health related issues. One of the most important aspects of medical caregiving is developing good relationships with doctors and other health-care professionals.

In the past, doctors typically took the lead and patients simply followed. Today, a good patient-doctor relationship (especially for eldercare) is more of a partnership between patient, family and doctor; all working together to solve medical problems and maintain good health. This means that you or your loved one should ask questions if the doctor's explanations or instructions are unclear, bring up problems even if the doctor doesn't ask, and let the doctor know when a treatment isn't working. If both you and your loved one take an active role in care, you will significantly decrease the chances of medical error and increase the odds that your loved one will receive the proper care and treatment.

Before you and your loved one visit the doctor's office, take some time together to prepare. Preparation increases your loved one's chances of leaving the appointment well-informed and satisfied with the care received.

If your loved one is visiting the doctor because he or she isn't feeling well, write down everything that both of you can remember about your loved one's symptoms, including what the symptoms are, how long they've lasted, and whether or not anyone else in the family has ever experienced similar symptoms. The more specific your loved one can be, the more he or she will help the doctor make an accurate diagnosis.

If your loved one is visiting the doctor for a routine checkup, write down any changes in his or her condition since the last doctor's visit, and any questions you both may have. You may want to find out, for example, whether or not your loved one should get a flu shot, or how often he or she should have a breast or prostate exam.

Also make sure that your loved one is prepared to tell the doctor about all the medications that he or she takes, including over-the-counter drugs, vitamins, and other supplements. Write down all the relevant information, including the dosage of each pill and how often your loved one takes it. Or you may simply want to take your loved one's medications — in their original containers — to the appointment.

The worksheets in this chapter can help you with many aspects of health care, from finding and evaluating a physician in the first place to managing medications and keeping track of doctor's appointments.

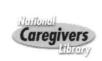

NOTES

DATE OF ENTRY	

Choosing the Right Doctor

If your loved one doesn't already have a primary physician—or if he or she is unhappy with the current doctor—the following kinds of questions can help you evaluate different physicians.

1. Has a consumer group rated doctors in the area where your loved one lives?

2. Does the doctor accept your loved one's health insurance?

3. In what areas does the doctor specialize? Do these areas match your loved one's needs?

4. Length of time in practice?

5. Where did the doctor receive his or her degrees and training?

6. Which hospitals does the doctor use?

7. What are the office hours?

8. Does the doctor speak the language you and your loved one are most comfortable speaking?

9. How many other doctors "cover" for the doctor when he or she is not available? Who are they?

10. How long does it usually take to get a routine appointment?

11. What happens if you need to cancel an appointment? Will you have to pay for it?

12. Does the office send reminders about prevention tests?

13. What do you do if your loved one has an "after hours" emergency?

14. Does the doctor give advice over the phone?

NOTES

DATE OF ENTRY	

15. Is the doctor aware of relevant community resources?

16. How long or difficult is the trip to the office? Is parking convenient?

17. If possible, accompany your loved one on his or her first visit. Did the doctor:

    a) Give you and your loved one a chance to ask questions?

    b) Really listen to *your* questions?

    c) Answer in terms you both understood?

    d) Show respect for you and your loved one?

    e) Ask you both questions?

    f) Make you both feel comfortable? Spend enough time with you?

    g) Address the health problem(s) your loved one came with?

    h) Ask about treatment preferences?

When evaluating a doctor, trust your own reactions but also give the relationship some time to develop. It will take more than one visit for you to get to know each other. Keep in mind:

- Give information. Don't wait to be asked.

- You know important things about your loved one's symptoms and health history. Tell the doctor what you think he or she needs to know.

- It is important to tell the doctor personal information—even if it makes you feel embarrassed or uncomfortable.

- Take your loved one's "health history" list with you (and keep it up to date).

- Make sure the doctor is aware of any medicines your loved one is taking. Talk about any allergies or reactions to medicines.

- Bring other medical information, such as x-ray films, test results, and medical records (or have them sent electronically).

- Ask questions. If you don't, the doctor may think you understand everything that was said.

- Write down questions before your visit. List the most important ones first to make sure they get asked and answered.

- **Take notes. Ask the doctor to repeat and explain anything you do not understand!!!**

94

NOTES

DATE OF ENTRY	

Appointment Information

If you are primarily responsible for your loved one's care, it will be important for you to keep detailed notes during doctor's appointments and make sure that you follow the doctor's instructions. Make a copy of this **Appointment Information** form before each examination and use it to keep track of any advice the doctor offers for your loved one's care.

Appointment Date/Time: _____

With:_____

Where:_____

Phone:_____

Reason for Appointment:_____

_____

Insurance Coverage or Payment Method for this Visit: _____

_____

_____

Changes in Condition? Treatment Progress? _____

_____

_____

_____

Procedures/Tests Performed? Results? New Tests Scheduled? Time, Date, Location of these tests?

_____

_____

_____

_____

NOTES

DATE OF ENTRY	

Outcomes from Current Medication? New Medication? Reason for Prescription? Side Effects?

_____

_____

_____

_____

_____

Support Services Recommended? Name, Address, Phone? _____

_____

_____

_____

_____

Referrals? Names, Addresses, Phone Numbers?:_____

_____

_____

_____

Next Appointment:_____

NOTES

DATE OF ENTRY	

Personal Health History

This worksheet can help generate a complete picture of your loved one's past and present medical condition. This is especially important if he or she is seeing a new doctor—or more than one doctor—because the information recorded in this form can alert health professionals to complications that might come from previous conditions or medications.

Full Name: ....

Date of Birth: ....

I was in the hospital for (list condition):

....Date: ....

....Date: ....

....Date: ....

....Date: ....

I have had these surgeries:

....Date: ....

....Date: ....

....Date: ....

....Date: ....

I have had these injuries/conditions/illnesses:

....Date: ....

....Date: ....

....Date: ....

....Date: ....

NOTES

DATE OF ENTRY	

I have these allergies:_____

_____

_____

Immunizations:	Suggested age:	Date received:
Influenza	Every year starting at 65	_____
Pneumococcal	Once at age 65	_____
Tetanus (Td)	Every 10 years	_____

I take the following medicines / supplements:

_____

_____

_____

_____

_____

My family members (parents, brothers, sisters, grandparents) have had these major conditions:

_____

_____

_____

_____

I see these healthcare providers: (List providers' names and conditions treated)

_____

_____

_____

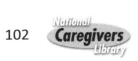

NOTES

DATE OF ENTRY	

Weekly Medicine Record

Make multiple copies of the larger Weekly Medicine Record (on page 105) to help your loved one keep track of which medicines to take on which days and when to take them. Also, use the chart to track that the medicine was actually taken.

Weekly Medicine Record

Name: _____

Week of: _____

Name & Dosage	Size, Shape, Color of Pill	When to Take Medicine	Sun	Mon	Tue	Wed	Thu	Fri	Sat

Write name and date, starting on Sunday, at the top of the record.

Each row is for one dose of medicine. Take the name and dosage of each medicine from the label on each container and write them under the first column. *For example: Lanoxin .25mg.*

In the second column, write the size, shape and color of the pill. *For example: Small, round, white pill.*

In the third column, write when to take the medicine. *For example: Before breakfast.*

When your loved one takes a medicine, place an "X" in the column for the day of the week. If your loved one takes a medicine more than once a day, mark it each time.

NOTES

DATE OF ENTRY	

Weekly Medicine Record

NOTE: Make multiple copies of this chart before writing. Save this original as a blank chart.

(You are hereby granted permission to make multiple copies of this chart for your own, personal, non-commercial use.)

Name: _____

Week Of: _____

Name & Dosage	Size, Shape, Color of Pill	When to Take Medicine	Sun	Mon	Tue	Wed	Thu	Fri	Sat

NOTES

DATE OF ENTRY	

Chapter 5: Legal Matters

Caregiving often involves handling a loved one's legal affairs. These can range from making or updating a will to signing advance medical directives or granting power of attorney.

You might begin by discussing your loved one's will or estate plans. The goal of estate planning is to distribute a person's assets and minimize taxes at death. For most of us, that means making and periodically updating a will. Also, various types of trusts or gifts can be arranged to help preserve assets for heirs. Trusts require the help of an attorney experienced in tax issues and estate planning. If your loved one hasn't made a will, discuss the importance of doing so and suggest setting up an appointment with an attorney.

Consider a durable power of attorney. This is a legal document giving one or more people the authority to handle finances, property, or other personal matters for another.

> *"Of all the documents anybody signs, a durable power of attorney could be the most important, especially for someone 55 or older," says Thomas D. Begley Jr., an elder law attorney in Moorestown, N.J. "It means that if you become incompetent you will have a person of your choosing ready to make decisions on your behalf, and it costs $100 instead of the $3,000 or more that it takes to have a guardian appointed by a court."*

However, a durable power of attorney may not neatly address all situations, so check with your lawyer about additional strategies for your family's particular situation.

Take a look at advance medical directives. If permitted by state law, most people should have a legal document that specifies the type of medical care they want or don't want if they become hopelessly ill and unable to communicate their wishes. Two good resources to learn more about advance directives are our website and the National Healthcare Decisions Day website at www.nhdd.org.

Experts recommend a "health care power of attorney" or "health care proxy," which designates a family member to make decisions about medical treatment and can provide guidelines for doing so. Among the reasons for health care proxies: they can prevent unwanted, unnecessary, and costly medical procedures.

Since **the specific laws regulating such matters vary from state to state**, you'll need to contact an attorney to handle the details. The worksheets in this chapter, however, can help get you pointed in the right direction.

NOTES

DATE OF ENTRY	

Evaluating Attorneys

An elder law attorney may be a good idea in cases involving seniors because these lawyers deal almost exclusively with the elderly and have a greater understanding of the specific issues and limitations that these individuals face.

Elder law attorneys typically specialize in a variety of areas including one or more of the following:

- Medicaid or Medicare claims and appeals

- Social Security and disability claims and appeals

- Supplemental and long-term health insurance issues

- Disability planning (i.e., durable power of attorney, living trusts, living wills, etc.)

- Conservatorships and guardianships

- Estate planning, including wills, probate, and trusts

- Administration and management of trusts and estates

- Long-term care placement

- Nursing home issues such as patient's rights and nursing home quality

- Elder abuse

- Housing issues (including age discrimination)

- Retirement, including public and private retirement benefits and pension benefits

Following are questions that you might ask any attorney when trying to decide if he or she is right for you and your loved one. Try asking these questions to several attorneys, and compare their answers before making a final decision.

1. How many attorneys are in the office that relate to the types of expertise you might need?

2. Who will handle your case?

3. If a trial is involved, does this same attorney do trial work?

NOTES

DATE OF ENTRY	

4. Is the attorney a member of the local bar association?

5. Will you be meeting with this attorney during your initial meeting?

6. How long has the attorney been in practice?

7. What type(s) of law does he or she specialize in?

8. How long has he or she been in this/these field(s)?

9. What percentage of his or her practice does he or she devote to each type of law?

10. Is there a fee for the first consultation and if so, how much?

11. Does the attorney bill differently for work that office paralegals or clerks do on your case?

12. What does the attorney charge for out-of-pocket costs?

13. How frequently does the attorney bill?

14. Would the attorney require a retainer in your case?

15. Would you be required to sign a contract?

16. Can an estimated fee for services be given?

17. Given the nature of your problem, what information should you have at the initial consultation?

During your meeting it is a good idea to ask:

18. What are my alternatives?

19. What are the advantages/disadvantages to each possibility?

After deciding on a course of action, ask your attorney for this in writing. Be sure to keep a copy of this in your files. Additionally, make sure that you understand what is required of you to help the attorney work on your case.

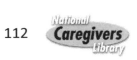

NOTES

DATE OF ENTRY	

Document Organizer

One of the biggest tasks you may face is finding and organizing all of your loved one's important paperwork. The **Document Organizer** can help you identify which legal, financial, and medical records you need to locate, and it provides a framework for keeping track of these documents for future reference.

This form can help you identify and locate the important documents you will need as a primary caregiver. There are six sections: **Health Care, Military, Identification, Financial, Insurance** and **End-of-Life Planning**.

Check "yes" or "no" to indicate whether or not you can put your hands on the document when needed. For every "no" (or if the document needs to be up-dated), write its name on a "to do" list and work to locate, create or revise these important papers.

Your loved one's current legal name: _____

Maiden or other name(s): _____

Health Care

❑ YES ❑ NO **Personal Medical Information and Health History**

This includes a listing of the names and phone numbers of doctors, a summary of the care recipient's medical history, and information about the health of immediate family members.

Document Location: _____
Primary Care Physician and Phone: _____

❑ YES ❑ NO **List of Current Medications**
For each medication, include the name, dosage, frequency and time of day, special instructions, prescription number, and physician. *NOTE: This list may change frequently. Keep it up to date.*

Document Location: _____
Pharmacy and Phone: _____

Military Records

❑ YES ❑ NO **Military Records**

Military ID Number: _____
Discharge Certificate. _____

Location of Documents: _____

114

NOTES

DATE OF ENTRY	

Identification

❑ YES ❑ NO   **Identity Records Folder**

Identification numbers should be guarded and given out only when a situation demands it. However, there may be circumstances when the primary caregiver must have proof of the care recipient's identity. Gather photocopies of the following documents and keep in a single, protected location.

Location of Identity Records: _____

❑ YES ❑ NO   **Social Security Card.** Number _____
❑ YES ❑ NO   **Driver's License.** Number_____
❑ YES ❑ NO   **Birth Certificate.**
❑ YES ❑ NO   **Marriage License(s).**
❑ YES ❑ NO   **Divorce Record(s).**
❑ YES ❑ NO   **Spouse's Death Certificate.**
❑ YES ❑ NO   **Adoption Certificate.**
❑ YES ❑ NO   **Naturalization Papers.**

Financial

❑ YES ❑ NO   **Financial Assets Inventory**
This is a master listing of the care recipient's assets showing account numbers and type, name and location of the financial institution, and contact name and phone numbers. This inventory should also account for property owned and any sources of income due the care recipient.

Location of Financial Assets Inventory: _____

❑ YES ❑ NO   **Checking Accounts**
These may be held by banks, credit unions, or brokerage houses and may take the form of standard checking or Money Market accounts.

❑ YES ❑ NO   **Savings Instruments**
Many people use multiple types of savings instruments, including regular savings accounts, Certificates of Deposit, and savings bonds.

❑ YES ❑ NO   **Investments**
Investment vehicles include publicly traded stocks and bonds, shares of mutual funds, IRAs, Keogh plans, and 401-K plans, etc.

❑ YES ❑ NO   **Sources of Revenue**
The care recipient may have funds coming from an employer (or business if self-employed) from wages or retirement plan, from Social Security, pension plans, annuity contracts, military retirement benefits, other government programs, tax refund, insurance claim or settlement, and the like.

NOTES

DATE OF ENTRY	

❏ YES ❏ NO **Real Estate Owned**

Includes independent or joint ownership of primary and secondary residence, vacation property (or time share), rental property, commercial property or vacant land.

❏ YES ❏ NO **Personal Property Owned**

These include automobiles and other vehicles, antiques and collections, and jewelry.

❏ YES ❏ NO **Inventory of Money Owed**

This is a master listing of debts showing the account number; the name and location of the financial institution; and a contact name and phone number. A checklist of items that go into this inventory includes:

- Mortgages
- Home Equity Loans
- Automobile Loans or Leases
- Other Secured Loans
- Business Loans (if self-employed)
- Unsecured Loans
- Credit Card Debt

❏ YES ❏ NO **Deed to House / Other Property**

Document Location: _____

❏ YES ❏ NO **Automobile / Vehicle Titles** (Auto, truck, motorcycle, trailers, etc.)

Document Location: _____

❏ YES ❏ NO **Loan Agreements**

Document Location: _____

❏ YES ❏ NO **Personal Property Appraisals** (jewelry, antiques, collections)

Document Location: _____

❏ YES ❏ NO **Tax Records**

Document Location: _____
Accountant's Name & Phone: _____

❏ YES ❏ NO **Veterans Benefits Documentation**

Document Location: _____
Contact Phone No. _____

NOTES

DATE OF ENTRY	

Insurance

❏ YES ❏ NO **Insurance Coverage Worksheet**
This is a master listing of all of the care recipient's insurance coverage showing: the policy numbers; the amounts of coverage; name of the company, company contact and phone; premium amount and due dates; and beneficiary.

Location of All Insurance Documents: ....

❏ YES ❏ NO **Life Insurance**
Includes multiple policies and types of insurance (group, whole life, term life, universal life, etc.).

❏ YES ❏ NO **Health Insurance**
Multiple sources of coverage are common, including a Health Insurance Supplement, Medigap policy, or Major Medical benefits.

❏ YES ❏ NO **Disability Insurance**

❏ YES ❏ NO **Long-term Care Insurance**

❏ YES ❏ NO **Homeowner's / Renter's Insurance**

❏ YES ❏ NO **Vehicle Insurance**
Many folks have multiple vehicles of various types, including recreational vehicles (RVs, campers, boats). Be sure to account for each.

❏ YES ❏ NO **Liability Insurance** (Personal, Business and/or Professional).

End-of-Life Planning

❏ YES ❏ NO **Last Will and Testament and Final Instructions**
Have circumstances changed? Does the care recipient want to make any revisions?

Location: ....
Attorney's Name & Phone: ....

❏ YES ❏ NO **Advance Medical Directives**
Has the care recipient signed a living will or other medical directive?

Document Location: ....

❏ YES ❏ NO **Burial Policy / Ownership Certificate for Cemetery Plot**

Document Location: ....

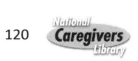

NOTES

DATE OF ENTRY	

Making a Will

The most basic and essential part of estate planning is a will. Yet, more than 60 percent of people never take the time to write one, leaving families confused and facing potential legal entanglements. While specific laws vary, this checklist offers general guidelines that apply in almost all cases. Use this as a starting point and make notes about your loved one's wishes before you sit down with an attorney.

> *NOTE: Your loved one's desires concerning medical care should be left out of the will, because this document is usually not read until after a death. Specific healthcare wishes belong in an Advance Medical Directive.*

A will:

- Should be prepared by a lawyer, on behalf of anyone over the age of 18.

- Should be double-checked when new laws or changing circumstances may affect the distribution of property.

- May need to be redrafted if an accident or sudden illness makes a family member something less than self-sufficient or solvent.

- May need to be revised when the value of property changes substantially.

- Should be checked for revisions after the birth of children or grandchildren, after a divorce, after a death in the family.

- Should name alternate beneficiaries.

- Should be checked for validity after moving to another state.

- Should substitute a new executor or personal representative if the one named can no longer serve.

- Can be used to name legal guardians.

- Should be placed in a fireproof safe or other secure place.

- Should not be placed in a safe deposit box unless the executor has joint access, although the box may certainly contain a copy.

- Should be drawn up while the maker is in good health and free from emotional stress.

NOTES

DATE OF ENTRY	

Chapter 6: Financial Caregiving

Understanding your loved one's finances—especially those of an aging parent—can be an incredibly important part of your caregiving role. But how do you ask a loved one to turn over checkbooks, credit cards, and savings to you if you suspect that he or she is having difficulty managing money?

Try to remember two things: (1) you know your loved one best and (2) always respect your loved one's safety and wishes.

Because you know your loved one best, you know the best way to approach him or her regarding money. In some cases, it may be easier to ask straight out if help is needed. But if your loved one is reluctant to discuss such matters, it may be better to hint at a financial conversation by speaking about your own finances. It may also be helpful to have a trusted advisor bring this up to your loved one. This might be their attorney, accountant, minister, rabbi, doctor or a close friend.

Regardless of how you approach the topic, remember that money allows individuals to be independent. This means that your loved one should have as much of a say as possible. By respecting your loved one in this manner, you will facilitate his or her continued independence.

- Make sure that your loved one understands that you're willing to help. It's better to offer help too soon than to let your loved one's finances fall into disarray.

- Listen for cues that suggest your loved one is asking for help (e.g., you are given a list of his or her bank accounts, you see a disorderly stack of unpaid bills on the counter, you hear him or her worry about not being able to meet financial needs).

Above all, unless your loved one lacks the capacity of judgment, always respect his or her financial decisions. If you are working on your own finances, offer to look into any questions your loved one may have.

Let your loved one know specifically what you need to be able to help manage his or her finances. The following worksheets can help get you started.

NOTES

DATE OF ENTRY	

Choosing a Financial Planner

Managing money can be a time-consuming and overwhelming task, so many people turn to Certified Financial Planners. A financial expert may be able to help you get organized and come up with a plan to pay for necessary care. If you and your loved one want to hire such a professional, use this worksheet to help you evaluate and choose the one who's right for you.

- How long has this individual been in practice? What types of clients does he or she typically work with? How are their situations similar to your loved one's?

- Does this person have experience in insurance, taxes, investments, estate planning?

- What kinds of credentials does he or she have? What about professional certifications?

- What is his or her educational background? What about former professional experience?

- What services are offered? Does the planner simply offer advice, or does he or she sell financial products as well?

- What is his or her philosophy when it comes to investing? Will this person carry out recommendations or refer you to someone else (attorneys, tax agents, insurance specialists)?

- Who else will work with you? How many clients and employees does the planner have?

- How is the planner paid? By the hour? A flat fee for services? On commission?

- Ask for a cost estimate, based on your loved one's situation and what is required. How much do these services typically cost? How long will the process take?

- Will you be able to put the plan into effect without retaining the planner's ongoing services?

- What companies also stand to benefit from the planner's recommendations? Is this individual "tied" to certain groups or financial products?

- Ask for a sample plan for another client facing some of the same issues.

- What does the planner want to know about your loved one's situation? How specific are his or her questions? What do they recommend?

- Which organizations regulate the planner? Has this person ever been disciplined by state insurance or securities departments or the Certified Financial Planner Association?

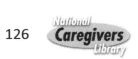

NOTES

DATE OF ENTRY	

Health Costs Estimator

Look at your loved one's medical and insurance records from the last year or two. Use them as guides to determine what services he or she might use this year. Check the first column of this form for services used, then list amounts covered under the policy and estimate the out-of-pocket expense for each service your loved one might need.

After totaling expenses, you may be able to decide whether you need to explore alternatives to pay for necessary care.

Services	Amount Covered By Insurance	Out of Pocket Expense
Hospital care		
Surgery (inpatient and outpatient)		
Office visits to your doctor		
Immunizations		
Mammograms		
X-Rays		
Mental health care		
Dental care and cleaning		
Vision care, eyeglasses and exams		
Prescription drugs		
Home health care		
Nursing home care		
Other services (list below):		
TOTAL:		

NOTES

DATE OF ENTRY	

Payment Options Chart

Caregiving can be expensive, and one of the biggest obstacles you and your loved one may face is simply finding a way to pay for necessary care and services. This chart offers a comparison of four different government programs, with emphasis on which services are covered by each.

NOTE: The chart may not cover every case possible and should be used only as a reference tool for discussing your pay options with a local qualified professional. **Government regulations change often. This chart is only a rough guide. Contact the appropriate agency to determine if these rules still apply.**

	Medicare	Medicaid	Medigap	Veteran's Benefits
Adult Day Care	No	Some states offer Medicaid	No	Some veteran's hospitals
Assisted Living	No	Coverage depends on type of care and	No	No
Care Management	No	Will not cover any private services or consultants.	No	Check with Veteran's Administration. Strict financial requirements apply.
Home Care	Only part-time or intermittent through certified agencies.	Yes, but length of coverage and type of services varies state by state.	Only when receiving skilled home care through Medicare.	Depends on availability in your area. Check with VA office and hospitals.*
Hospice	Yes, contingent on doctor's diagnosis of terminal illness and hospice certification.	Yes, contingent on doctor's diagnosis of terminal illness and hospice certification.	No	May be offered in some VA hospitals or by VA affiliated home health care.

(Continued on page 131)

NOTES

DATE OF ENTRY	

Payment Options Chart - continued

	Medicare	Medicaid	Medigap	Veteran's Benefits
Housekeeping	No	Some states offer waivers for funding limited services	No	Depends on VA home care unit and services in your area.
Nursing Home	Pays for 20 days in skilled nursing facility. Significant per day co-pay after 20 days. All coverage stops after 100 days. Does not cover custodial care.	Covers most costs, but only at facilities offering a lower rate. Choice of facilities is very limited, as are types of care services.	Some plans offer "skilled nursing co-insurance" to help defray costs not covered by Medicare.	Some VA facilities offer long-term skilled nursing and intermediate care. Rare instances of custodial care.
Respite Care	No	No	Varies by state. Contact Area Agency on Aging.	Depends on VA home care unit and services in your area.
Support Groups	No	No	No	Contact VA hospital or clinic.
Transportation	No	No	No	Very limited reimbursement for travel to VA medical care.

* May extend to spouses, widows, or dependents of veterans.

NOTES

DATE OF ENTRY	

Alternative Ways of Financing Care

After exploring standard payment methods, you may need to consider alternative sources of money, including:

- Living Benefits (from an existing life insurance policy)
- Viaticals
- Reverse Mortgages

Living benefits are proceeds, usually 25 to 100 percent of the death benefit, from life insurance policies that may be paid before death. Conditions under which these payments are made are very specific.

- To determine if your loved one's life insurance policy offers advance payment alternatives, call the state insurance commission or check with the insurance company's claims department. Ask whether your loved one's policy pays these benefits and how much they cost.

- Accelerated benefits are sometimes added to policies for an additional premium, usually computed as a percentage of the base premium. Some companies offer the benefits at no extra premium, but charge for the option when it is used.

- The company will almost always reduce the benefits advanced to the policyholder before death to compensate for interest lost on the early payout. There may also be a service charge.

Viaticals refer to the purchase of a life insurance policy for a percentage of the policy's face value.

Reverse Mortgages. If your loved one owns a home, you might want to consider a reverse mortgage (RM). Reverse mortgages can be a very good source of cash for your loved one and there are many reputable companies offering them. However, consulting with an attorney or financial advisor before making this decision is essential.

There are three kinds of RMs: Federal Housing Authority (FHA)-Insured, Lender-Insured, and Uninsured. Each type varies, but there are some features most RMs have in common:

- They are rising-debt loans with interest added to the principal each month.

- RMs charge origination fees and closing costs. Insured plans may involve insurance premiums.

- RMs use up equity in a home, leaving your loved one with fewer assets.

- The initial loan advance at closing may be negotiated higher than the rest of the payments made to the homeowner.

- Legal obligation to pay back the loan is limited by the value of the home at the time of repayment. This could include increases in the home's appreciation after the loan begins.

- RM loan advances are non-taxable and do not affect Social Security or Medicare benefits.

NOTES

DATE OF ENTRY	

Chapter 7: End-of-Life Planning

If you have been placed into an end-of-life caregiving role by a crisis or event, try not to second-guess what you are feeling. Understand that conflicting emotions – fear, anger, grief, and helplessness—are natural, and have confidence in your own judgment.

Trust Yourself

Trust in your ability to handle these additional responsibilities, but also realize that some things are out of your control. If you feel yourself losing perspective, consider talking with a faith leader or counselor.

Having some knowledge about what lies ahead – physically, emotionally, and spiritually – can make a real difference as you and your family prepare for the death of your loved one. Talk to your loved one's doctor, nurse, and other members of the health care team about what to expect. Discuss these issues with family members, friends, children, and visitors when appropriate.

Connect with support structures

This includes family, friends, clergy and ministers, professionals, volunteers – anyone and everyone who has something to offer. Take advantage of help wherever you can find it, and avoid the all-too-common tendency of caregivers to become isolated.

Keep in mind, too, that most people want to help, but may be uncomfortable making the offer or with the circumstances. Make it easier for them, by letting them know what they can do, in a concrete, practical way.

Review legal and financial arrangements

This may include wills, powers of attorney (both financial and healthcare), "no code" or do-not-resuscitate orders, as well as the location and disposition of important documents and proofs of ownership. Having all of these measures in place and up-to-date will spare you and your family time and difficulty.

Maintain your health and well-being

It's easy to lose sight of your own needs and requirements during this time. Do what you can to maintain balance in your own life—physically, spiritually, and socially. If you feel selfish or guilty for spending time on yourself, keep in mind that no one can draw water from an empty well.

NOTES

DATE OF ENTRY	

Evaluate hospice

Hospice shifts the goal of treatment from healing to dying with dignity. Hospice services have a high success rate in easing pain and helping terminal patients remain comfortable. Some families have a difficult time with the idea of stopping efforts to combat a disease, but it's important to consider all options. Because the hospice team (which includes physicians, nurses, social workers, counselors, clergy, therapists, and volunteers) will work closely with your loved one – and the rest of the family – to help them through the experience of dying, you may want to interview services in advance and choose a group that everyone feels comfortable with.

"Palliative care" programs likewise focus on maintaining comfort, but there is no expectation that life-prolonging therapies will not be used. And while hospice services commonly take place in the home, palliative care teams usually work in facilities or institutions.

Pre-plan if you can

There are many steps that can and should be taken well in advance of a loved one's final days. These include a letter of last instructions (in which your loved one sets down his or her wishes for the funeral or ceremony), as well as pre-planning with a funeral home.

This can be one of the most difficult responsibilities that many caregivers face. If possible, you and your loved one should discuss such matters far ahead of time, when everyone is calm and thinking clearly. This offers the additional reassurance that matters are being carried out in accordance with your loved one's wishes.

The checklists found in this section can help make this very difficult responsibility a little bit easier.

- Hospice shifts the goal of treatment from healing to dying with dignity, easing pain, and helping terminal patients remain comfortable. Because the hospice team (which includes physicians, nurses, social workers, counselors, clergy, therapists, and volunteers), will work closely with the family to help them through the end-of-life process, you may want to interview services in advance and choose a group that everyone feels comfortable with. Use the **Hospice Questions** form as you evaluate various services.

- The **Funeral Planning Form** can help you and/or your loved one finalize the details of his or her memorial service and burial. Ideally, this form would be completed by your loved one ahead of time, so he or she could specify his or her wishes. But the form can help guide you through the process regardless of the specifics of the situation.

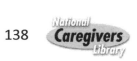

NOTES

DATE OF ENTRY	

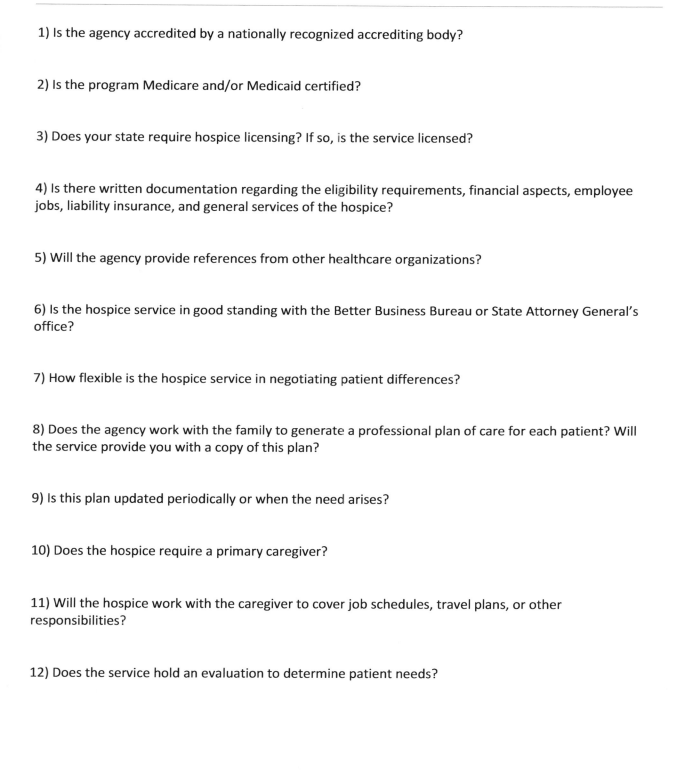

Questions About Hospice Care

1) Is the agency accredited by a nationally recognized accrediting body?

2) Is the program Medicare and/or Medicaid certified?

3) Does your state require hospice licensing? If so, is the service licensed?

4) Is there written documentation regarding the eligibility requirements, financial aspects, employee jobs, liability insurance, and general services of the hospice?

5) Will the agency provide references from other healthcare organizations?

6) Is the hospice service in good standing with the Better Business Bureau or State Attorney General's office?

7) How flexible is the hospice service in negotiating patient differences?

8) Does the agency work with the family to generate a professional plan of care for each patient? Will the service provide you with a copy of this plan?

9) Is this plan updated periodically or when the need arises?

10) Does the hospice require a primary caregiver?

11) Will the hospice work with the caregiver to cover job schedules, travel plans, or other responsibilities?

12) Does the service hold an evaluation to determine patient needs?

NOTES

DATE OF ENTRY	

13) Does the service consider what the patient can do for him or herself?

14) How many personnel references does the agency require?

15) Are the hospice workers licensed and bonded?

16) Does the agency have a routine way of handling complaints?

17) How does the agency handle billing?

18) Will the agency help find financial assistance?

19) Are there payment plans available?

20) Does the agency have a 24 hour on-call service?

21) How quickly do hospice services begin?

22) What specialized services are available?

23) What are the policies regarding residential admission? Inpatient care? Which hospitals work closely with the residential facilities?

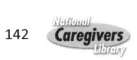

NOTES

DATE OF ENTRY	

Funeral Planning Form

As your loved one makes his or her funeral plans, use this form to record all of his or her wishes for final arrangements.

Final Arrangements for:_____

Memorial Services
Funeral home:
Funeral director:
Location of service:
To be officiated by:
Military/fraternal/social organization or lodge members to be present:
Pallbearers:
Veteran's flag: ❑ Folded ❑ Draped on casket
Music:
Reading or scripture selections:
Flowers: ❑ Yes ❑ No
Memorial donations: ❑ Yes ❑ No
Name of charitable organization:
Casket: ❑ Open ❑ Closed **OR** Cremated remains present? ❑ Yes ❑ No
Preparation and printing of the order of memorial services (sometimes provided as part of service by funeral director with assistance from family):

NOTES

DATE OF ENTRY	

Burial

Name, address, and phone of cemetery:

Cemetery documents located:

Casket: ❑ Wood ❑ Bronze ❑ Copper ❑ Steel

Burial Vault (usually required by cemetery/may be purchased through funeral home or cemetery—check on pricing):

Property or crypt purchased? ❑ Yes ❑ No

Location:

No. of spaces:

Type of burial: ❑ Earth burial ❑ Crypt ❑ Mausoleum ❑ Other:

Inscription to read:

Other information or instructions:

Cremation

Name, address, and phone number of funeral home or cremation society:

Urn: ❑ Bronze ❑ Wooden ❑ Marble ❑ Other:

Location of cremated remains: Cemetery Private estate

Final Disposition: ❑ Earth Burial ❑ Mausoleum ❑ Crypt ❑ Columbarium ❑ Other:

Alternative disposition:

Type of memorial or monument:

Inscription:

NOTES

DATE OF ENTRY	

On a separate sheet of paper, make a record of the following information

Preparing An Obituary:
Name of deceased:
Spouse's name:
Date and place of death:
Children/cities where they reside:
Grandchildren/cities where they reside:
Siblings/cities where they reside:
Parents/cities where they reside (or resided, if deceased):
Date, time, and place of funeral or memorial service and burial:
Clergy/person officiating:
Address of funeral home: Address of cemetery:
Memorial contributions may be made in lieu of flowers to: (optional)
Photo preferred:
Place and date of birth:
Education:
Wedding date:
Military service:
Employment:
Religious affiliation: Other Affiliations:
Significant achievements:

NOTES

DATE OF ENTRY	

About the Author

Ron Moore founded Office America, one of the first office supply superstore chains. Office America grew to more than 20 stores and over $70 million in sales before Staples acquired it. Moore also created the Supply Room Companies, an office products business that has grown to over $50 million in sales by following a "roll-up" and consolidation strategy.

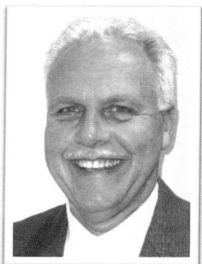

As an independent consultant to Circuit City, the former electronics-retailing giant, Moore identified the opportunity to create the first used car superstore concept, which became CarMax (KMX) in 1993. CarMax surged to $1 billion in annual sales, faster than companies like Home Depot, Wal-Mart and McDonalds, and currently has sales in excess of $15 billion annually.

Moore provides opportunity identification, strategy development, new venture creation, and other corporate development services to clients ranging from individuals and family firms to Fortune 500 companies and non-profit organizations. His primary areas of expertise include:

Analyzing trends and identifying major opportunities that others have missed.
- Generating conceptual possibilities and analyzing them strategically.
- Understanding consumer cognition to discover new ways of reaching and doing business with customers.
- Creating new ventures
- Executing merger, acquisition and divestiture strategies.

Focusing his skills on the implications of the Aging of America, Moore has become a recognized leader in identifying ways that the *age wave* and the *caregiving phenomenon* create both opportunities and threats for companies in virtually every industry, from healthcare to financial services to real estate, construction, retail, transportation, and technology.

Moore combined his professional expertise with his personal experiences in dealing with the difficulties and dynamics of caring for aging parents to create the National Caregivers Library, a national resource for caregivers, the organizations to whom they turn for help and companies that offer products and services to them.

Keynote Speeches, Executive Briefings and Presentations

Caregiving has heated up as an important employer issue. Major organizations—even governments— are recognizing the tremendous costs and productivity drains on employers caused by workers dealing with caregiving issues. And, they are asking why employers have not done more already to address these issues and what can be done about it.

Moore is often asked to address these problems and to discuss ideas on how to get employers more engaged in providing solutions to the expanding number of working caregivers.

A frequent speaker on opportunity identification and the impact of the aging of America in the marketplace, in the workplace and on the home front, Moore has lectured at numerous colleges, universities, and business and professional organizations. Among them are the University of Richmond, Virginia Commonwealth University, The College of William & Mary, Virginia Tech; chapters of the National Association of Women Business Owners (NAWBO), The Family Business Forum, the National Association of Healthcare Executives and numerous AARP and government conferences.

Moore was a lead speaker at the national conference of the Rosalynn Carter Institute and a leading witness to the California Senate Subcommittee on Aging and Long Term Care where he addressed *Caregiving as a workplace issue*—what corporate America can do to help caregiving employees and improve bottom-line operating results. His keynote address to the Ohio Governor's Conference on Aging presented a business case for why employers must seek solutions to the challenges and costs of an aging population and workforce. Moore has also been an adjunct professor at Virginia Commonwealth University, where he led a graduate course on Opportunity Identification in an Aging Society.

Topic specialties include:

- Aging in America: Problem or Opportunity?
- Aging, Caregiving and Corporate America
- The Business Case for Eldercare / Caregiving Programs in the Workplace
- Opportunity Identification and the Implications of an Aging Society
- Opportunities for the Faith Community in an Aging Society
- New Venture Creation - for businesses, non-profits and churches

Moore is a graduate of Hampden-Sydney College in Virginia. He resides in Richmond and serves on several Boards and Advisory Committees, including Virginia Blood Services, the Department of Gerontology at Virginia Commonwealth University and others, and he is active in his church.

Sources

In addition to consulting with professionals in the areas of geriatric care management, elder law, aging-in-place, gerontology, hospice, funeral planning and other pertinent disciplines, the publisher utilized the following sources while creating the Caregivers Workbook.

Chapter One
"Caregiver's Assessment Worksheet" adapted from "Elder Care Choices and Decisions: Locating Community Resources," B3603-2, produced by University of Wisconsin-Extension Cooperative Extension Services and the U.S. Department of Agriculture 1995; and the *Care Manager's for Caregivers Project* developed by the Rosalynn Carter Institute 2001. Adapted and used with permission.

"Taking Care of Yourself" adapted from materials originally developed by the Aging and Adult Services Administration Department of Social and Health Services, State of Washington. Adapted and used with permission

"Problem-Solving Worksheet" adapted from "Elder Care Choices and Decisions: Caring For the Caregiver," B3603-5, produced by the University of Wisconsin-Extension Cooperative Extension Services in conjunction with the U.S. Department of Agriculture, 1995.

Statistics provided by "Family Caregiving in the U.S.," by the National Alliance for Caregiving, Bethesda, MD and The American Association of Retired Person, Washington, DC .

Chapter Two
Introduction adapted from "Providing Day-to-Day Care," originally written and published by the Aging and Adult Services Administration Department of Social and Health Services, State of Washington. Adapted and used with permission.

"Home Care Workers" adapted from "Elder Action: Action Ideas For Older Persons and Their Families." *Caregivers, Caregiving and Home Care Workers,* developed by the Administration on Aging.

"Home Safety Checklist" adapted from materials originally created by the U.S. Consumer Product Safety Commission and materials originally written and published by the Aging and Adult Services Administration Department of Social and Health Services, State of Washington. Adapted and used with permission. Also, consulted for "Home Safety Checklist": "Elder Action: Action Ideas for Older Persons and Their Families." *Home Modification and Repair* prepared by the Administration on Aging from materials developed by the National Eldercare Institute on Housing and Supportive Services, Andrus Gerontology Center, University of Southern California.

Chapter Three
"Questions for Assisted Living" adapted and used with permission. from materials produced by the Consumer Cooperative on Assisted Living.

"Nursing Home checklist" adapted from "Your Guide to Choosing a Nursing Home," United States Department of Health and Human Services Health Care Financing Administration.

Chapter Four
Introduction adapted from "Talking With Your Doctor: A Guide For Older People," developed by the United States National Institutes of Health National Institute on Aging.

"Choosing the Right Doctor" adapted from "Choosing a Doctor. Your Guide to Choosing Quality Health Care," developed by the Agency for Health Care Policy and Research (AHCPR), in cooperation with other agencies of the U.S. Department of Health and Human Services.

"Personal Health History" adapted from materials developed by the National Institutes of Health. "Weekly Medicine Record" adapted from "Living With Heart Disease: Is It Heart Failure?" AHCPR Publication No. 94-0614, developed by the United States Agency for Health Care Policy and Research.

Chapter Five
Introduction adapted from "Financial Caregiving: A Survival Guide." *FDIC Consumer News.*, Federal Deposit Insurance Corporation; and *The DOD Caregiver's Guide* developed by the United States Department of Defense.

Chapter Six
"Choosing a Financial Planner" adapted from "Choosing a Financial Planner," G93-1163-A, produced by the University of Nebraska Cooperative Extension Services in cooperation with the United States Department of Agriculture.

Chapter Seven
Developed in cooperation with Blair Nelsen, owner of Nelsen Funeral Homes, Richmond, VA.

Made in the USA
Lexington, KY
05 July 2018